INSULIN RESISTANCE DIET

WHAT TO EAT AND WHY

Dr, Tiffany J. Bozeman

CONTENT

INTRODUCTION

People's awareness of insulin resistance, which happens when body cells become resistant to the actions of insulin and raise blood sugar levels, is becoming more and more important for their health. While medicine is a treatment option for insulin resistance, lifestyle modifications like nutrition are also a viable alternative for managing it. Concerning the insulin resistance diet, this book seeks to give readers a complete how-to manual that explains both what to eat and why.

CHAPTER ONE

Insulin Resistance: An Overview

High blood sugar levels are a result of the condition known as insulin resistance, which interferes with the body's capacity to utilize insulin properly. By enabling cells to utilize glucose for energy, the hormone insulin, which is generated by the pancreas, aids in controlling blood sugar levels. An accumulation of glucose in the circulation occurs when the body develops an inability to utilize insulin, which makes it resistant to it.

What exactly is insulin resistance?

As cells in the body lose their sensitivity to the effects of insulin, it leads to high blood glucose levels. This condition is known as insulin resistance. Since the body cannot correctly manage blood sugar levels, this disease frequently results in prediabetes or type 2 diabetes.

To make up for insulin resistance, the pancreas increases insulin production. Yet, with time, the pancreas may not be able to keep up with the body's needs, resulting in excessive blood sugar levels and other health issues.

What Leads to Insulin Resistance?

Insulin resistance can occur as a result of several circumstances, such as:

1. Genetics: Certain individuals may have a hereditary predisposition to insulin resistance, increasing the likelihood of developing the illness.

2. Obesity: Excess body fat, particularly in the belly, might raise the chance of developing insulin resistance.

3. Sedentary Lifestyle: A sedentary lifestyle and a lack of exercise might raise the risk of insulin resistance.

4. Unhealthy Diet: A diet rich in sugary and processed foods might raise the chance of developing insulin resistance.

5. Age: Insulin resistance risk rises with advancing age.

Diagnosis and Symptoms

Many people may not be aware they have insulin resistance until it results in prediabetes or type 2 diabetes since it frequently has no symptoms. Nonetheless, some individuals may display signs like:

1. Tiredness
2. mental fog
3. Growing hunger
4. Weight loss challenges
5. Elevated blood sugar

A doctor may do several tests to identify insulin resistance, including:

1. An eight-hour fast is required for the fasting blood sugar test, which evaluates blood sugar levels.

2. Oral glucose tolerance test: In this test, blood sugar levels are monitored over time after consuming a sweet solution.

3. The hemoglobin A1c test evaluates blood sugar levels on average over the previous two to three months.

Diabetes and Insulin Resistance: Effects

Some negative effects of insulin resistance include:

1. Type 2 diabetes: Type 2 diabetes, a chronic illness that affects millions of individuals worldwide, is one of the primary causes of insulin resistance.

2. Cardiovascular Disease: Blood arteries can be damaged by high blood sugar levels, which increases the risk of heart disease and stroke.

3. Polycystic Ovary Syndrome: Polycystic ovary syndrome (PCOS), a disorder that

affects the ovaries and can lead to infertility and other health issues, can develop as a result of insulin resistance.

4. Nonalcoholic Fatty Liver Disease: Nonalcoholic fatty liver disease (NAFLD), a disorder that causes the liver to retain too much fat, can be exacerbated by insulin resistance.

5. Sleep Apnea: Insulin resistance may raise the chance of developing sleep apnea, which interferes with breathing while you're asleep.

To treat this illness and avoid its effects, it is essential to comprehend insulin resistance. Reduced risk of insulin resistance and the health issues it is connected with can be achieved with a nutritious diet, consistent exercise, and other lifestyle modifications.

CHAPTER TWO

Dietary Factors Affecting Insulin Resistance

Genetics, exercise, food, and other variables can all have an impact on insulin resistance, which is a complicated disorder.

To manage insulin resistance, a balanced diet is essential since it can impact the body's capacity to control blood sugar levels.

Diet's Impact on Insulin Resistance

The onset and treatment of insulin resistance are significantly influenced by diet. A diet heavy in whole foods, fiber, and healthy fats can assist improve insulin sensitivity and blood sugar management whereas a diet high in processed foods, refined carbs, and saturated fats can contribute to insulin resistance.

An Important Dietary Balance

For the management of insulin resistance, a balanced diet is necessary. The risk of type 2 diabetes can be decreased by eating a diet high in fruits, vegetables, whole grains, lean protein, and healthy fats. On the other hand, a diet heavy in refined carbs added sugars, and saturated and trans fats can cause insulin resistance, weight gain, and other health issues.

What Macronutrients Do

1. Carbohydrates, proteins, and fats are the three primary nutrients in the diet. Each macronutrient has a unique physiological function and has the potential to influence insulin sensitivity in various ways.

2. Protein: Protein is necessary for the development and maintenance of

muscular tissue and helps control blood sugar levels. A high-protein diet has been demonstrated in studies to increase insulin sensitivity and lower the risk of type 2 diabetes.

3. Fats: Beneficial fats, such as mono- and polyunsaturated fats, can help increase insulin sensitivity and lessen inflammation in the body. Yet, an excessive intake of saturated and trans fats in the diet can lead to insulin resistance and other health issues.

4. Carbohydrates: The body's primary fuel source, carbohydrates also have an impact on insulin sensitivity. Insulin

resistance and a higher risk of type 2 diabetes can result from a diet heavy in refined carbohydrates, such as white bread and sugary beverages.

A diet high in complex carbs, on the other hand, can enhance insulin sensitivity and lower the risk of type 2 diabetes. These foods include whole grains, fruits, and vegetables.

Carbohydrates' Effect on Insulin Resistance

As carbohydrates are the body's primary supply of glucose, they can significantly affect insulin resistance. To assist get glucose from the circulation into the cells for energy, insulin is generated when carbs are broken down into glucose. Yet, an excessive intake of refined carbohydrates might cause insulin resistance because the body becomes less responsive to the effects of insulin.

The speedy conversion of simple carbs like sugar and white bread into glucose causes a sharp rise in blood sugar levels. Large levels of insulin may be released as a result, eventually resulting in insulin resistance. Complex carbs, on the other hand, including those found in whole grains, fruits, and vegetables, break down more gradually, resulting in a slower rise in blood sugar levels and a decreased need for insulin.

Improved insulin sensitivity and a decreased risk of type 2 diabetes can both be achieved by eating a diet high in complex carbs, fiber, and whole foods. A high-fiber diet has been linked to improved insulin sensitivity and blood sugar regulation, whereas a low-fiber diet has been linked to weight gain and insulin resistance.

Diet plays a critical role in treating insulin resistance and reducing the health issues that come with it. Improved insulin sensitivity and blood sugar management can be achieved with a well-balanced diet full of whole foods, fiber, lean protein, and healthy fats. Those who want to control insulin resistance and lower their risk of type 2 diabetes can make educated dietary decisions if they are aware of the effects of macronutrients, especially carbs.

CHAPTER THREE

What to Eat if You Have Insulin Resistance

Focusing on nutrient-dense, whole foods that are high in fiber, lean protein, healthy fats, and complex carbs is the key to an insulin resistance diet. The items to include in an insulin-resistance diet that can enhance insulin sensitivity, control blood sugar levels, and lower the risk of type 2 diabetes are covered in this chapter.

Nutritional Carbohydrates

Given that they give the body nutrition and energy, healthy carbohydrates are crucial in an insulin resistance diet. Nevertheless, complex carbs should always be chosen above refined carbohydrates as they are digested more gradually and do not result in sharp rises in blood sugar levels.

On an insulin resistance diet, you can eat some types of healthful carbs, like:

1. Whole grains are a great source of minerals, fiber, and complex carbs. This includes whole wheat, oats, quinoa, and brown rice.

2. Fruits: Fruits are a great source of fiber, nutrients, and vitamins. For people with insulin resistance, low-glycemic fruits including berries, apples, and pears are ideal options.

3. Vegetables: Vegetables are abundant in fiber, vitamins, and minerals while being low in calories. For an insulin resistance diet, leafy greens, cruciferous veggies, and root vegetables are all excellent options.

Foods High in Fiber

As fiber slows down the absorption of glucose into circulation, which helps control blood sugar levels, fiber is crucial in treating insulin resistance. Moreover, fiber encourages satiety, which might assist those with insulin resistance in controlling their weight.

Include the following fiber-rich foods in your diet if you have insulin resistance:

1. Whole grains are a fantastic source of fiber, vitamins, and minerals.

2. Legumes: Beans, lentils, and peas are nutrient- and fiber-rich.
3. Vegetables and fruits: Vegetables and fruits are full of fiber and other necessary elements.

Healthy proteins

Protein is crucial for the development and maintenance of muscular tissue, and it also has the potential to control blood sugar levels. For those with insulin resistance, lean proteins are the ideal option since they are low in saturated fats, which can exacerbate insulin resistance and other health issues.

Lean proteins that can be incorporated into an insulin resistance diet include:

1. Fish: Omega-3 fatty acids, which are abundant in fatty fish like salmon, mackerel, and sardines, can enhance

insulin sensitivity and lessen inflammation.

2. Poultry: Great sources of lean protein include chicken and turkey.

3. Legumes: Peas, beans, and lentils are high in fiber and protein.

Suitable Fats

An insulin resistance diet must include healthy fats like monounsaturated and polyunsaturated fats since they can increase insulin sensitivity and decrease inflammation. Saturated and trans fats should be avoided nevertheless because they have been linked to insulin resistance and other health issues.

Here are some illustrations of good fats to incorporate into an insulin resistance diet:

1. Avocado: An wonderful source of fiber, monounsaturated fats, and other necessary nutrients is avocado.

Almonds, walnuts, chia seeds, and flaxseeds are full of fiber, protein, and healthy fats.
3. Fatty fish: Fish high in omega-3 fatty acids, such as salmon, mackerel, and sardines, might enhance insulin sensitivity and lessen inflammation.

Vitamin-Rich Foods

An insulin resistance diet must include foods high in antioxidants since they can help lower oxidative stress and inflammation, two factors that can lead to insulin resistance and other health issues. Examples of foods high in antioxidants that can be incorporated into an insulin resistance diet include:

1. Berries: Strawberries, blueberries, and raspberries are high in fiber and antioxidants.

2. Dark chocolate: Due to its high antioxidant content, dark chocolate

might enhance insulin sensitivity and lessen inflammation.

The third option is green tea.

CHAPTER FOUR

Diets for Insulin Resistance: Foods to Avoid

Nutrient-dense, whole foods that are low in sugar, processed carbs, and harmful fats should be the mainstay of an insulin resistance diet. The foods to avoid on an insulin resistance diet that might cause insulin resistance, inflammation, and other health issues are covered in this chapter.

Basic Carbohydrates

Simple carbs readily convert to glucose, resulting in sharp increases in blood sugar levels. Insulin resistance and associated health issues including type 2 diabetes, obesity, and heart disease may result from this. With an insulin resistance diet, simple carbs should be avoided including:

1. White pasta, rice, and bread
2. Sweetened cereals
3. Sweets and candies
4. Baked products, including pastries, cookies, and cakes

Finished Products

Processed foods are generally deficient in nutrients and excessive in sugar, salt, and harmful fats. They can aggravate inflammation, insulin resistance, and other medical conditions. While following an insulin resistance diet, avoid processed foods like:

1. Quick meals
2.2. Frozen food
3. crackers and chips
4. packaged snacks like protein and granola bars

Fattening Foods

Foods with a lot of fat, especially those with a lot of saturated and trans fats, might worsen insulin resistance and other health issues. These lipids can disrupt insulin signaling and lead to inflammation. Avoid these high-fat items while following an insulin resistance diet:

1. Fries and fried chicken are examples of fried cuisine.

2. Meats high in fat, such as bacon, and sausage

3. dairy items with added fat, such as cheese and ice cream
4. Margarine with butter

Sugary Drinks

Sugar-rich drinks including soda, fruit juice, and sports drinks might exacerbate insulin resistance and other medical conditions. These beverages include a lot of sugar and can quickly raise blood sugar levels. With an insulin resistance diet, you should avoid sugar-sweetened beverages like:

1. Sodas and energy beverages
2. Fruit beverage
3. Sweetened coffee and tea beverages
4. Sports beverages

Alcohol

Alcohol can affect insulin signaling and make you more likely to develop insulin resistance. Inflammation and other medical conditions including liver disease and high blood pressure can also be exacerbated by it. If you're on an insulin resistance diet, you should restrict or avoid alcohol.

1. Beer

Cocktails and sweet wines

3. Mixtures of distilled alcohol and sweet mixers

Nutrient-dense, whole foods that are low in sugar, processed carbs, and harmful fats should be the mainstay of an insulin resistance diet. For those with insulin resistance, limiting simple carbs, processed meals, high-fat foods, sugary drinks, and alcohol can increase insulin sensitivity, control blood sugar levels,

and lower the risk of type 2 diabetes and
other health issues.

CHAPTER FIVE

Planning And Preparing Meals

For those with insulin resistance, a nutritious and balanced diet is crucial to controlling blood sugar levels, increasing insulin sensitivity, and lowering the risk of type 2 diabetes and other health issues.

Advice on Food Preparation

1. Emphasize nutrient-dense, whole foods: People with insulin resistance should eat a balanced diet that includes a range of nutrient-dense, whole foods

such as fruits, vegetables, lean proteins, healthy fats, and complex carbs.

2. Choose foods with a low glycemic index: These foods can help control blood sugar levels and enhance insulin sensitivity. Whole grains, legumes, non-starchy vegetables, and certain fruits are foods with a low glycemic index.

3. Strive for well-balanced meals: For those with insulin resistance, a well-balanced meal should contain a supply of protein, complex carbs, and healthy fats.

4. Manage portion sizes: Maintaining healthy blood sugar levels and avoiding overeating are made possible by managing portion sizes.

5. Maintain hydration: Staying hydrated and drinking enough water will help control blood sugar levels and prevent dehydration.

a sample menu for people with insulin resistance

Breakfast

1. A cooked egg on a slice of whole-grain bread with avocado
2. A cup of berry-mixed fruit.

3. 1 cup of almond milk without added sugar

Snack:

1. A single tiny apple and one spoonful of almond butter.

Lunch

1. Roasted veggies and grilled chicken breast (carrots, zucchini, and bell peppers)
2. A half-cup of quinoa
3. 1 cup of green tea without sugar

Snack

1. 1 cup of hummus and cucumber slices

Dinner

1. Baked salmon with brown rice and steamed broccoli
2. One little sweet potato.
3. 1 cup of herbal tea without sugar

Tips for Preparing Meals

1. Prepare meals ahead of time: Making meals ahead of time can save time and help avoid the temptation of bad foods.

2. Employ nutritious cooking techniques: Nutrients may be retained and harmful

fats can be avoided by using nutritious cooking techniques including grilling, baking, steaming, and roasting.

3. Make use of healthy foods: Lean proteins, low-fat dairy products, herbs, and spices as well as olive oil are examples of nutritious components.

4. Manage portion proportions: To manage portion sizes and prevent overeating, use measuring cups and food scales.

Snack Concepts

1. Greek yogurt and a selection of fruit
2. Hummus and raw veggies

3. carrot sticks with a hard-boiled egg

4. Almond butter with apple slices

5. A smoothie made with spinach, mixed berries, and unsweetened almond milk.

To control blood sugar levels, increase insulin sensitivity, and lower the risk of type 2 diabetes, and other health issues, people with insulin resistance must plan and prepare their meals. People with insulin resistance can maintain a healthy and balanced diet by adhering to meal planning advice, utilizing healthy foods and cooking techniques, and managing portion sizes. Including healthy snack options can also help you avoid overeating and the lure of junk food.

CHAPTER SIX

Modifying Your Lifestyle to Control Insulin Resistance

A large part in addressing insulin resistance can be played by lifestyle modifications in addition to nutrition. This chapter will cover several lifestyle modifications that people with insulin resistance can do to enhance their well-being and lower their chance of contracting type 2 diabetes and other illnesses.

Physical Activity and Workout

For those with insulin resistance to manage their disease, regular exercise and physical activity are essential. Exercise can help reduce weight growth, manage blood sugar levels, and increase insulin sensitivity. A minimum of 150 minutes of moderate-intensity aerobic activity or 75 minutes of vigorous-intensity aerobic activity is advised for those with insulin resistance week.

Cycling, swimming, dancing, and brisk walking are a few examples of moderate-intensity aerobic exercise. Running, high-intensity interval training and sports like basketball or soccer are all examples of vigorous-intensity aerobic activity.

Insulin-resistant people might potentially benefit from strength training activities like weightlifting or resistance band workouts. Muscle mass may be increased by strength training, which enhances insulin sensitivity and controls blood sugar levels.

Strategies for Managing Stress

Blood sugar levels and insulin resistance can both suffer from prolonged stress. Using stress-reduction strategies like yoga, deep breathing, meditation, or frequent massages might help lower stress levels and enhance insulin sensitivity.

Reading, listening to music, having a warm bath, and other relaxation practices can all help lower stress levels.

Making Time for Sleep

For those with insulin resistance, getting enough sleep is essential. Lack of sleep can impact insulin sensitivity, boost hunger, and cause weight gain. Adults should attempt to get at least 7-8 hours of sleep each night.

To enhance the quality of their sleep, people with insomnia or other sleep problems should consult a doctor.

Other Lifestyle Modifications to Control Insulin Resistance

There are further lifestyle modifications that people with insulin resistance can make in addition to exercise, stress reduction, and sufficient rest to manage their condition:

1. Drink in moderation: Alcohol intake can influence blood sugar levels and raise the risk of weight gain. Men should restrict their daily alcohol intake to no

more than two drinks, while women should limit their daily alcohol intake to no more than one drink.

2. Give up smoking: Smoking raises the risk of type 2 diabetes and insulin resistance. Improved insulin sensitivity and a decreased risk of various health issues can both be a result of quitting smoking.

3. Maintain hydration: Staying hydrated and drinking enough water will help control blood sugar levels and prevent dehydration.

4. Minimize sedentary activity to assist increase insulin sensitivity and lower the risk of weight gain. Sedentary behavior includes things like sitting for extended periods. It is advised that people take regular breaks and move about throughout the day.

The management of insulin resistance can be greatly aided by lifestyle modifications such as regular exercise, stress reduction strategies, enough sleep, moderation in alcohol use, stopping smoking, maintaining hydration, and lowering sedentary behavior. Individuals with insulin resistance can enhance their health, lower their chance of becoming type 2 diabetes, and avoid other health issues by making certain lifestyle adjustments. Before making any major lifestyle changes, it is advised that people speak with a healthcare provider.